The Beginners Guide To Kegel Exercises

A Complete Beginners Guide To Kegel Exercises; Doubling Strength Gains 7x And Strategies For Achieving Bodybuilding Goals

Vicky Klocko

Table of Contents

CHAPTER ONE 3
- Kegel Exercises 3
- Understanding Pelvic Floor Muscles 5
- Performing Kegel Exercises 7
- Benefits of Kegel Exercises 12

CHAPTER TWO 16
- Incorporating Kegel Exercises 16
- Tips for Consistency 17
- Advanced Tips 19
- Advanced Kegel Techniques 20

CHAPTER THREE 26
- Pregnancy and Postpartum Benefits 26
- Benefits for Men's Health 27
- Lifestyle and Pelvic Health 29
- Long-Term Benefits of Kegel Exercises 31
- Embracing Kegel Exercises for Well-Being 32
- Conclusion 33

THE END 37

CHAPTER ONE

Kegel Exercises

Kegel exercises are a series of exercises designed to strengthen the pelvic floor muscles. These muscles support the bladder, uterus, rectum, and intestines. The exercises involve contracting and relaxing the pelvic floor muscles repeatedly to improve their strength and endurance.

Kegel exercises are often recommended for various reasons:

Urinary incontinence: Strengthening these muscles can help prevent or reduce leakage of urine.

Postpartum recovery: Women often perform Kegel exercises after childbirth to regain pelvic floor strength.

Improved sexual function: Strengthening these muscles can potentially enhance sexual satisfaction for both men and women.

To perform Kegel exercises, you contract the pelvic floor muscles (the ones used to stop the flow of urine) for a few seconds, then relax them for the same duration. It's essential to do these exercises regularly to see improvement.

Understanding Pelvic Floor Muscles

Understanding the pelvic floor muscles is crucial for understanding the significance of pelvic health.

The pelvic floor is a group of muscles that forms a supportive sling at the base of the pelvis. These muscles play a vital role in various functions:

Support: They support the pelvic organs, including the bladder, uterus, and rectum. A strong pelvic floor provides stability and prevents these organs from descending or prolapsing.

Urinary and Bowel Control: The pelvic floor muscles work in coordination with the urinary and anal sphincters to control the release of urine and feces. Weak pelvic floor muscles can lead to urinary or fecal incontinence.

Sexual Function: These muscles are involved in sexual function, including arousal and orgasm. Strengthening them can enhance sexual sensation and satisfaction.

Maintaining good pelvic health is essential for overall well-being. Factors such as pregnancy and childbirth, aging, obesity, chronic coughing, and certain surgeries can weaken the pelvic floor muscles. Weakness in these muscles can lead to issues like urinary incontinence, pelvic organ prolapse, and diminished sexual function.

Performing Kegel Exercises

Performing Kegel exercises involves correctly identifying and engaging the pelvic floor muscles. Here's how to do it and execute the exercises correctly:

Identifying Pelvic Floor Muscles:

Stop the Flow: When you urinate, try to stop the flow of urine midstream. The muscles you use to do this are your pelvic floor muscles. However, don't make a habit of regularly stopping your urine flow, as it can disrupt bladder emptying and may lead to issues.

Squeeze and Lift: Another way to identify the pelvic floor muscles is to imagine stopping passing gas by contracting the muscles around the anus and vagina (for both men and women). You should feel a pulling sensation or a lift upward.

Correct Kegel Exercise Technique:

Find a Comfortable Position: You can perform Kegel exercises lying down, sitting, or standing—whichever is most comfortable for you.

Contract the Muscles: Once you've identified the pelvic floor muscles, contract them by squeezing and lifting upward. Try not to tighten your abdomen, thighs, or buttocks during this contraction.

Hold and Release: Hold the contraction for about 3-5 seconds at first. As you get more comfortable, gradually increase the duration up to 10 seconds. Then, relax the muscles for an equal amount of time. This relaxation phase is as crucial as the contraction.

Repeat and Schedule: Aim for 10-15 repetitions, 3 times a day. Remember, consistency is key. You can incorporate these exercises into your daily routine, like doing them while watching TV or during regular daily activities.

Avoid Overdoing It: Don't overwork the muscles by doing too many Kegels at once, as this can lead to muscle fatigue.

Breathe Normally: Maintain normal breathing throughout the exercise. Don't hold your breath.

Be Patient: Results may take time. It can take a few weeks to a few months of regular practice to notice improvements in pelvic floor strength.

Benefits of Kegel Exercises

Kegel exercises offer numerous benefits, particularly in enhancing bladder control and improving overall pelvic health.

For Enhancing Bladder Control:

Reducing Urinary Incontinence: Strengthening the pelvic floor muscles can help prevent or reduce instances of urinary incontinence, including stress incontinence (leakage when coughing, sneezing, or laughing) and urge incontinence (sudden strong urges to urinate).

Postpartum Recovery: Women who perform Kegel exercises after childbirth often experience faster recovery of bladder control and pelvic floor strength.

For Improving Pelvic Health:

Preventing Pelvic Organ Prolapse: A strong pelvic floor provides support to pelvic organs. Strengthening these muscles can help prevent or reduce the risk of pelvic organ prolapse, where organs like the bladder, uterus, or rectum descend into the vagina.

Enhanced Sexual Function: Improved pelvic floor strength can lead to increased sexual sensation and satisfaction for both men and women. Stronger muscles can contribute to better control and potentially more intense orgasms.

Improved Posture and Stability: Strong pelvic floor muscles contribute to better core strength, which aids in maintaining good posture and stability.**Preventing Other Complications:** Strong pelvic floor muscles can help prevent complications associated with weak pelvic support, such as back pain or discomfort.

CHAPTER TWO

Incorporating Kegel Exercises

Incorporating Kegel exercises into your routine can be straightforward with a few simple steps and consistency:

Establishing a Kegel Routine:

Set Reminders: Set specific times throughout your day to perform Kegel exercises. It could be after waking up, during breaks at work, or before going to bed.

Routine Integration: Associate Kegels with daily activities. For instance, do them while brushing your teeth, waiting at a traffic signal, or during TV commercials.

Journaling or Apps: Use a journal or apps to track your progress and remind yourself of your exercise routine. Some apps provide reminders and structured workout plans for Kegels.

Tips for Consistency

Start Slow: Begin with a manageable number of repetitions and gradually increase over time. Consistency is more important than intensity when starting.

Make it a Habit: Incorporate Kegel exercises into your daily habits, just like brushing your teeth or having meals. Consistency will make them feel like a natural part of your routine.

Be Patient: Results take time. Don't be discouraged if you don't notice immediate changes. Consistent practice over weeks or months often yields significant improvements.

Find What Works for You: Experiment with different positions and times of day to find when and where you're most comfortable doing Kegels.

Accountability Partner: Share your goal of incorporating Kegel exercises with a friend or partner. This accountability can help you stay motivated.

Advanced Tips

Progressive Training: As your pelvic floor muscles get stronger, increase the duration of each contraction and the number of repetitions. Gradually challenge yourself for continued improvement.

Combine with Other Exercises: Pair Kegel exercises with other routines, like yoga or Pilates that focus on core strength and flexibility.

By establishing a routine and incorporating these exercises into your daily life, you can improve consistency and maximize the benefits of Kegel exercises for bladder control and pelvic health. Remember, consistency is key, so finding ways to make these exercises a regular part of your day will yield the best results.

Advanced Kegel Techniques

Advancing your Kegel exercises involves gradual progression and exploring variations to increase strength and effectiveness. Here are some advanced techniques:

Gradual Progression:

Extended Contractions: Start by gradually increasing the duration of each contraction. Begin with 3-5 seconds and work your way up to 10 seconds or longer if comfortable.

Increased Repetitions: As your muscles strengthen, aim to increase the number of repetitions in each session. Gradually add more repetitions, but avoid overexertion.

Resistance Training: Use Kegel balls or resistance devices specifically designed for pelvic floor exercises.

These can add resistance and challenge your muscles for improved strength.

Variations for Increased Strength:

Elevated Positions: Try performing Kegels in different positions like standing, squatting, or on your hands and knees. These variations engage the muscles differently and can intensify the workout.

Dual Focus: Combine Kegel exercises with other movements. For instance, while doing squats or lunges, engage your pelvic floor muscles simultaneously.

Quick Contractions (Flutter Kegels):
Alternate between rapid contractions and relaxations of the pelvic floor muscles. This technique can enhance muscle responsiveness.

Mixed Durations: Incorporate a mix of short and long contractions within the same session. For example, alternate between 5-second and 10-second holds for variety.

Breath Control: Coordinate your breathing with the contractions. Inhale and relax the muscles, then exhale while contracting them. This synchronization can enhance muscle control and coordination.

Biofeedback Devices: Consider using biofeedback devices that provide real-time feedback on muscle activity. These tools can help you ensure you're engaging the correct muscles and measure your progress.

Caution:

Avoid Overexertion: Just like any exercise, avoid overworking the muscles. Listen to your body and don't push too hard, especially if you experience discomfort or pain.

Consult a Professional: If unsure about advanced techniques or if you have specific concerns, consult a pelvic floor physical therapist. They can guide you through tailored exercises based on your needs and progression level.

CHAPTER THREE
Pregnancy and Postpartum Benefits

Kegel exercises offer specific benefits for both pregnancy/postpartum and men's health:

Preparation for Childbirth: Performing Kegel exercises during pregnancy can strengthen pelvic floor muscles, which may help with the birthing process by improving muscle control and potentially reducing the risk of tearing.

Postpartum Recovery: After childbirth, Kegels can aid in the recovery of pelvic floor muscles that might have been strained or weakened during labor. They can assist in regaining bladder control and supporting pelvic organs.

Preventing or Reducing Incontinence: Strengthening the pelvic floor muscles during and after pregnancy can significantly reduce the likelihood of urinary incontinence that is common during and after childbirth.

Benefits for Men's Health

Improving Bladder Control: Kegel exercises can assist in managing and improving bladder control issues in men, especially those experiencing urinary incontinence due to prostate issues or other conditions.

Erectile Dysfunction (ED): Some research suggests that regular Kegel exercises can potentially aid in improving erectile function by strengthening the pelvic floor muscles involved in maintaining erections and ejaculatory control.

Prostate Health: After prostate surgery, men may experience urinary incontinence. Kegel exercises can be beneficial in regaining urinary control by strengthening the pelvic floor muscles.

Lifestyle and Pelvic Health

Lifestyle habits can significantly impact pelvic wellness, and incorporating Kegel exercises into your routine can yield long-term benefits for overall well-being:

Impact of Habits on Pelvic Wellness:

Physical Activity: Regular exercise contributes to overall health, including pelvic wellness. Engaging in activities that promote core strength, like yoga or

Pilates, can indirectly support pelvic floor health.

Healthy Weight Management: Maintaining a healthy weight reduces strain on the pelvic floor muscles. Excess weight can put pressure on these muscles, potentially leading to weakness and pelvic floor disorders.**Posture:** Good posture supports the pelvic region and reduces undue stress on the pelvic floor. Practices such as proper sitting and standing ergonomics can help in this regard.

Long-Term Benefits of Kegel Exercises

Prevention of Pelvic Issues: Consistent Kegel exercises can prevent pelvic floor disorders, such as urinary incontinence and pelvic organ prolapse, by strengthening the muscles that support these organs.

Improved Sexual Function: Strengthening pelvic floor muscles through Kegels can enhance sexual satisfaction by improving muscle tone and control.

Support Through Aging: Regularly practicing Kegel exercises can help maintain pelvic floor strength as you age, potentially reducing the risk of pelvic floor problems common in later years.

Embracing Kegel Exercises for Well-Being

Holistic Health Approach: Incorporating Kegel exercises into your routine promotes a holistic approach to health by addressing an often overlooked but vital aspect of overall wellness.**Self-Care and Empowerment:** Engaging in pelvic floor exercises like Kegels is a form of self-care and empowerment. It allows individuals to actively take charge of their pelvic health.

Confidence and Comfort: Strengthening pelvic floor muscles can enhance confidence and comfort in daily activities by reducing the likelihood of bladder leaks or discomfort.

Conclusion

The practice of Kegel exercises stands as a remarkable and accessible means of fostering pelvic wellness and overall well-being. By understanding and engaging the pelvic floor muscles through these exercises, individuals can experience a multitude of benefits.

From enhancing bladder control to fortifying pelvic health, the impact of Kegel exercises extends to various facets of life. For pregnant individuals, postpartum recovery can be supported, while men can find benefits in managing urinary concerns and aspects of sexual health.

The integration of Kegel exercises into daily routines becomes an empowering act of self-care. As consistency becomes a cornerstone, these exercises, alongside other healthy lifestyle habits, contribute to holistic well-being. They offer resilience against pelvic floor disorders, bolstering confidence and comfort in day-to-day activities.

Ultimately, embracing Kegel exercises signifies a proactive step toward personal wellness, underlining the significance of these exercises beyond their immediate benefits. With proper understanding, commitment, and integration into one's lifestyle, Kegel exercises stand as a testament to the transformative power of simple yet impactful practices in fostering long-term health and vitality.

THE END

www.ingramcontent.com/pod-product-compliance
Lightning Source LLC
Chambersburg PA
CBHW072049230526
45479CB00009B/333